YOGNOSIS
Core of Lore

Acharya Birju Maharaj

Copyright © 2018 Acharya Birju Maharaj

All rights reserved.

ISBN: 1983813591
ISBN-13: 978-1983813597

Important Notice: For Reasons of Legality

The author of this book, Acharya Birju Maharaj believes that the facts, figures, and knowledge presented herein should be available to every person concerned with improving his or her state of health. Although the author has attempted to give a profound understanding of the topics discussed and to ensure accuracy and completeness of any information that originates from any other source than his own, he and the publisher assume no responsibility for errors, inaccuracies, omissions, or any inconsistency herein. Any slights of people or organizations are unintentional. This book is not intended to replace the advice and treatment of a physician who specializes in the treatment of diseases. Any use of the information set forth herein is entirely at the reader's discretion. The author and publisher are not responsible for any adverse effects or consequences resulting from the use of any of the practice or procedures described in this book. The statements made herein are for educational and theoretical purposes only and are mainly based on Acharya Birju Maharaj's own experiences, opinions and theories. One should always consult a physician or a healthcare practitioner before taking up any of the practices or procedures mentioned herein this book. The author does not intent to provide any medical advice or offer a substitute thereof, and makes no warranty whatsoever, whether expressed or implied, with respect to any practice, procedure or therapy. Except as otherwise noted, no statement in this book has been reviewed or approved by any of the legal authority. Readers should use their own judgment or consult a holistic medical expert or their personal physician for specific applications to their individual problems. Author of this book have intentionally omitted mentioning literatures, links, justifications, expert quotes, research works done on Yoga or Yoga as therapy till date, as he does not want to create further confusion about Yoga as Therapy through this book. Author has tried to present the embedded facts about Yoga as the innate nature of Life within Nature and has thus intentionally omitted references and bibliographies presented on the subject till date. May some of the mentions of scriptures or articles relate to the presentations in this book as references or a coincidence! Information provided here are related to people residing in India and one shall not get confused with the same to be similar for other people in rest of the world.

DEDICATION

This Literature is dedicated to my Guruji His Holiness Brahmaleen Swami Manuvaryaji Maharaj.

I present this literature as a part of my endeavor to enlighten everyone on the globe with this inherent wisdom of Yoga as a wisdom of Nature for sound physical, mental, emotional and spiritual health and intrinsic cure.

- Acharya Birju Maharaj

PREFACE

'Yogic wisdom' reputedly possessed by the ancient Indian Gnostics (Seers and Rishis) who discovered the same to be essential to salvation from all ills or negatives of a Life; is termed thus as 'Yognosis'.

Hindu Samskriti is the epitome of wisdom acquired by Gnostics with their constant quest for healthy and blissful Life. Hindus acquired the highest level of evolution through their wisdom leading to best utilization of all creature comforts offered by Nature.

"Yoga neither is a belief system nor a science but the inherent wisdom of a creature to acquire higher levels of evolution to perfection that leads one to live an anticipated life for enjoyment of all the creature comforts offered by Nature and liberate from all bondages (limitations, Fear, Diseases, Disorders…) of life."

Yoga neither is a set of practices developed by Human though presented in such a manner by some people with individual identities from time to time, nor a religion. Yoga actually is the 'named identity' for inherent wisdom of an organism facilitating evolution and intrinsic mechanism to correct or say cure from within; May it be a unicellular organism or a well-developed human being. It may hurt many scholars who have done research in Yoga as Philosophy, Discipline and occult Science or as a Set of

Physical, Mental and Spiritual ritual. I shall clear all the doubts, ifs and buts in my explanations within this book. My efforts to unravel this Yogic wisdom of Nature to mankind is the duty of mine towards my Gurudev who dedicated entire of his life for the same purpose, to the larger benefits of the humanity.

Enormous amount of information and knowledge about health, illness and various measures to heal or cure are available hither and thither. There are numerous Scriptures describing Indian wisdom also available as manuscripts and also as printed literatures. None of them describes Yoga as an inherent operating system of Life that not only is the common platform or say bridge between Hardware and Software of Life developed by Nature, but has all the capacity to correct their malfunctioning; with intention or inadvertently.

Technological advancement has eased human life. Almost all the diseases of modern time are claimed to be cured completely by many systems of medicine yet failed to be as effective and precise as claimed. That is because human life is not like an instrument that if manufactured by one company, remains the same with all features similar for every individual throughout the world. Human life has evolved and not created! Human life has evolved to the highest level not because they are same, but because they all are different in almost all the aspects of life except their apparent gross physicality. Fixing a particular cracked bone will require almost the same skill for remedy anywhere in the world but subtle manifestation and the psyche of an individual that reflects in one's action, emotion, will, acceptance, level of understanding, belief, personality, health etc; needs an individualized approach and an exceptional expertise of a complete system of cure and this fact is of great significance for all including health professionals.

No wonder people throughout the globe are in the search of a cure for all diseases of present time, most of which are psychosomatic and lifestyle diseases for which they are left almost without cure. I have no prejudice for any system of medicine or methods of healing and would like to clear that all the systems of medicine are for the betterment of mankind and have their own significance as science of cure.

One needs to have a thorough understanding of the system applied to cure. The ambit and limitations of the system opted for cure needs to be verified primarily before opting them for healing or cure, not only because those are dealing with your body and many a times mind but most of the times damages caused by them remains irreversible and sometimes Fatal. There are two possible ways to cure. One is the intrinsic cure and other is extrinsic cure. The earlier uses prevalent inherent powers of an individual to cure a disease while the latter may use Natural resources, herbs, chemicals, derived bio-chemicals, basic elements and minerals, genetic modifications brought about from various sources and likewise. It is proven that intrinsic cure is the best way to cure among the two as is prevalent in each organism Naturally. As it is from within, intrinsic cure neither has side effects nor leads to further complications to a patient. Existence and evolution of the organism through millions of years is the evidence for the same and no further justifications shall be needed. Extrinsic cure on other hand can have side effects and most of the time leads to further or other complications. Intrinsic system of cure has a larger and empirical ambit of healing and cure. It largely has all the capacity to cure a disease with permanence from its root cause.

We all are victims of time based chronological belief systems on which we have to depend for knowing the most known and prevalent aspects of our life, one of which is Yoga. People from time to time believed Yoga to be a religion or a set of physical mental and spiritual regimes, a discipline for blissful life, Sacred practices for self-enlightenment and liberation, a Philosophy, a weapon or skill helping destroy enemies, a path to omniscience, process of raising and expansion of consciousness, an analysis of perception and cognition, a tradition and what not? What shall we believe what Yoga is? Shall we believe Śiva Yoga, Vedas, Upanishads, Śrutis, Darshan Shashtras like 'Samkhya' or 'Patanjali YogDarshan', Shrimad Bhagwad Gita, Hathyogpradeepika, Gherand Samhita, Yoga in Buddhism, Yoga in Jainism, Gyan Yoga, Bhakti Yoga, Karma Yoga, Raj Yoga, Hath Yoga, Laya Yoga, Natya Yoga, Naad Yoga, Kundalini Yoga and so many other forms known as Yoga? All these are confusing for an aspirant even with a micro-fine search! All these verses of literature though describes only Yoga, actually describes their own understanding and about the use of Yoga as an instrument or path within their desired disciplines and not actually innate Yoga!

In the path of evolution to perfection, human being acquired several beneficiary features for a perfect life and reached at the highest levels of perfection by recognizing and exploring the prevalent and inherent wisdom of Yoga offered by Nature. These advance features of life offered by Nature and acquired by human through the process of evolution includes expression of emotions, ability to design and frame the life as anticipated, making the best use of all the creature comforts offered by Nature, enjoy perfection and liberate from bondages like fear, sufferings, diseases, disorders etc.. A creature actually does not require any system of cure as all the creatures are endowed by Mother Nature with inherent capacity to stay healthy and cure itself from within. Yoga was not practiced or focused as therapy separately because this inherent wisdom of Life (named Yoga) was recognized by Yognostics (Great Indian Seers) and have had imbibed the same in the lifestyle of Indians long before the time of Vedas, and people were enjoying health and bliss because of this Yogic Lifestyle. Some people with ignorance about the same are wrongfully or may be intentionally mentioning Yoga as recently immerging system of Cure. Yoga Therapy (Yognosis) is not an immerging system of Cure but an inherent system of cure, as old as origin of Life.

There are several logical questions that really are more important for the logical and rational minds to satisfy entire of their quest about Yoga and to understand it as an inherent wisdom of Nature. According to all the scripture that includes Yoga as syllable or a theory of wisdom or a practice or a discipline; Śiva is the first fully evolved human at the time. He is known as Adiyogi (First Yogi), Adinath (First fully evolved human), Adishwar (Originator of life as first fully evolved human) and so on; and suppose if Yoga is a human creation, then how come Śiva knew Yoga? From whom Śiva learned Yoga? In which language Śiva shared his knowledge of Yoga with Śivani and Saptarishis? Did Śiva know Sanskrit, Prakrit or any other language? If yes, who taught him then? If Yoga is descended from him, then why there is a vast difference in descriptions of Yoga in different Scriptures? And so on.

Maharshi Patanjali answers such questions as an aphorism in his Yog Darshan,

"Bhava-pratyayo videha-prakriti-layanam"- P.Y.S.

"Some people are born with true insight (of Nature's wisdom, named Yoga) whereas others attain via a divine body (Guru, who is one with this insight) or oneness with Nature."

Maharshi Patanjali, through 'Yog Darshan' also have presented Yoga as an inherent wisdom of balanced life based on the Binary system of Nature and is not technically understood by any scholars of Yoga till date. Yoga scholars who are conversant with Yogic anatomy and physiology or medical science, if studies Yog Darshan or Samkhya Yoga as a practical Yoga guide to health and perfection in modern perspective, can easily understand the inherent binary wisdom of Yoga explained by Maharshi Patanjali.

"Tato Dwandwanabhighatah" – P.Y.S.

"Thus (with prevalence of Yoga in a Life) all inequalities (imbalances or disorders) those originate from Duality ends." or can be further explained as, "Thus it (Yoga) tends to mastery over the dual nature of life."

"Avidhya-ksetram-uttaresham-prasupta-tanu-vichchhinn-odaranam" – P.Y.S.

Ignorance (Avidhya) (lack of insight about being a born Yogi) is the source of most kleshās (diseases) that can be dormant, developing, developed, and devastating."

"Anitya-ashuchi-duhkha-anatmasunitya-shuchisukha-atmakhyatir-Avidhya" – P.Y.S."

An imbalance between the eternal and transitory, purity and impurity, joy and suffering, or the mutable and immutable in human beings are all referred to as a lack of insight (Avidhya – Root cause of Diseases/ Disorders)."

A creature is a born Yogi, but the fact is unknown to one. Enlightened ones of ancient times (Gnostics) discovered the prevalent wisdom in every living organism inherently provided by Nature for healing and evolution to perfection and named it 'Yoga' that operates life as the operating system. We have developed every solution for all the questions of life from and within this Operating System of life over the time through evolution.

Yoga is the operating system of life as needed in a

computer to function. Let us not make this operating system of life difficult to understand and occult but more comfortable to recognize and apply for the youth of today who are thriving for such wisdom that easily, instantly, effortlessly and intrinsically can correct life.

Human being though reached at the top of the evolution tree, has forgotten the continuum of Nature for evolution that inculcates the inherent capability to be perfect and heal oneself from within, and thus started suffering from many diseases and disorders. Ignorance about nature of Nature and being a born yogi who can design and direct one's life, who can best utilize the inherently acquired powers through the process of evolution to heal from within; leads to confusion and conflicts in one's mind that further manifest as the delusion of being diseased and finally turns diseased.

Unfortunately, many of such diseases are genetically adapted over the period of time through generations and expressed as Genetic Trait (Chitt Samskara) in the consequent progeny and preceded with permanence (Devastating).

With due respect to 'Tao-ism' (Yin-Yang) and 'Samkhya Darshan' (Purush-Prakriti) that are based on these principles of duality of Nature, I must say that principally both of the disciplines explained lately are correct and highly informative but practically short of applied techniques to use those for individual completeness or perfection and that is why their disciplines are understood as philosophies and not wisdom. Though one of the fellow disciple and scholar of Samkhya Philosophy namely Maharshi Patanjali described a systematized eight fold path of Yoga in his Yoga Sutras. Yoga remained only a discipline as those did not describe much on Methods or Techniques. Matsyendranath, Gorakshnath, Valmiki, Sandipani, Gherand muni, Swatmaram and many seers (Yognostics) described Yoga with some of the Practical Techniques that are practiced now a day in authentic schools of Yoga yet lacking the **core of Yogic lore.**

The entire universe is the manifestation of dual vibrating forces, wrapped into two great polarized energies (Purush and Prakriti or say Śiva and Śakti) that are interdependent though opposite and yet complementary to each other. The whole existence is reverberations of vibrating energy only.

We see duality at every aspect of life, wherever we look in nature, within ourselves or our mind. Moving from macrocosmic to microcosmic, gross to atomic, two great principles or forces can be seen at work balancing whole universe; may they be growth and degeneration, Day and Night, Sun and Moon, hot and cold, light and dark, positive and negative, male and female or there may be any other aspect. All other forces are the result of the playful manifestations of these primitive vibrating dual forces only.

Life is governed by the Binary System of Nature, that is named Śiva and Śakti, corresponding to the right nostril (Pinglā, Yang, Purush) and left nostril (Idā, Yin, Prakriti);

and to make it simple to understand, I have documented the inherent operating system of Life that is based on Binary System of Nature in this book that is named Yoga before thousands of years that can operate life with perfection as done with computers now a days. Nature has also provided us the ways to manipulate, modify and manage the operating system of life as Yoga, from within and also through Techniques derived by our ancestors to facilitate humans achieve desired results.

One who describes a universally unexplored theory or practice should not be confused to be the originator of the same. Maharshi Patanjali, a great Yogi of the time reconnoitered, described and systematized the wisdom of Yoga through 'Patanjali Yog Darshan'- literally means 'Exploration of the wisdom of Yoga in a distinctive way to canvas its prevalence and significance in a life". Maharshi Patanjali has beautifully and precisely explained Yoga and never claimed him-self to be an authority for invention, construction or origination of this Wisdom of Nature but presented a systematized and a useful way of application of the inherent Yogic wisdom and ancestral techniques based on this inherent wisdom for a blissful life, while many of others indoctrinated this inherent wisdom within day to day life performances of individuals as a doctrine for a jubilant life.

There are many paths of Yoga practiced till date and numbers of new forms are adding up every day. It is always confusing for aspirants about which path is to be followed. May it be Rajyoga, Hathyoga, Ashtang Yoga, Laya Yoga,

Dhyan Yoga, Vinyasa Yoga, Iyengar Yoga, Power Yoga, Hot Yoga, Ariel Yoga, Antigravity Yoga…and so on…and may be thousands more. I have experienced that Yoga is an ocean (Operating System) where all these faculties reach as rivers (Programs) and yet is the source of origin for all these rivers benefiting life. I have tried to present the complete ocean of inherent wisdom undivided into rivers of different faculties originating from it.

Inherent and profound Wisdom of Yoga had lost its dignity and profoundness due to different nomenclatures given from time to time to the wisdom of Yoga and such people without any role to play in have attached their name to the Wisdom of Yoga as a pioneer or architect or constructor or originator of this inherent Natural wisdom. While none of the oldest and original scriptures including Lord Śiva (Adi Yogi) have mentioned or attached any name as authority for pioneering, designing or inventing this Wisdom of Nature; many ignorants finding this as no man's land have attached their own or a different name with it to enjoy supremacy. That has canvassed Yoga a regional, religious, philosophical or spiritual practice that is thought to be devoid of any authentic wisdom behind it in the eyes of the people of modern era. Damage caused by these people to the inherent wisdom of Yoga is unforgivable and fatal.

Today, Yoga is considered only as a set of physical wellness practice that may prevent some of the Diseases and Disorders and nothing more. None of the so called authorities are accepting Yoga as an utmost technology inherently available to one contributing to complete health and healing from within.

Fortunately or unfortunately, research on Yoga is inspired by human doubts and uncertainty about knowing the Life and its characteristics to reason. A chemical or a drug and its effect on human body certainly require a thorough research as can work or harm adversely, but it is not appropriate to conduct such analytical research work on Yoga, as that is the intrinsic wisdom of Nature prevalent in every individual to overcome diseases and disorders and thus harmless. Thus, it is not at all necessary to conduct any analytical research on any of the faculty (including Yoga) of the wisdom of Nature that has created, maintained and evolved life including life of human being and that does not require any evidence for the same to be working in an anticipated manner! Will such research change the spirit of Nature or can we create a Nature based on our analytical research to convince our rational minds?

With all the respect for modern scientists who live their life for others and all medical practitioners saving lives on this planet, I would like to raise one question to all : "Aren't we becoming insane searching more external remedies by forgetting inherent powers and ancestral wisdom of healing, keeping and retrieving sound physical, mental and spiritual health?" Isn't it like a sailor trying to invent formulas of forming drinking water and investing all his efforts to invent a device or a gadget to produce drinking water for his and other companions' survival, overlooking that he is sailing in a drinking water lake!?"

There are number of diseases and traumatic conditions that need external remedial help for different reasons. May all modern medicine men focus on those conditions and put their efforts in that direction to save life and not on those which can be cured from within without much effort, obviously. Diseases of genetic trait in an individual are difficult to cure from within as the operating system of life (Yoga) fails to recognize it as a disease (Malware – Virus) and thus fails to trigger healing. Such and like diseases can be cured by researching Gene Therapy and like, should be of prime focus for researchers. Most of the diseases except few are psychosomatic and lifestyle diseases that can easily be cured by inherent and primitive wisdom for cure. History of modern medicine is not vast and people always found remedy for such lifestyle, self-acquired and manmade diseases through the inherent and primitive wisdom even before the birth of any system of Medicine.

Though humans have found almost all solutions for their day-to-day problems in life and have developed all the materials, instruments, and skills to ease life; still finds problems unsolved when it comes to Physiological, Emotional, Mental and Spiritual aspects of life. Yoga as an Operating System of life designed by Nature serves as great solution to such problems of an individual.

It is very easy now a day to understand human anatomy and physiology as described and understood in Yogic wisdom as it is similar to the structural and functional composition of a computer today. There are Nadis and Chakras for the regulation of energy (Prān) in the body as done in computers by circuits and logical gates (AND GATE and NAND GATE, OR GATE and NOR GATE, XOR GATE and XNOR GATE etc.) that regulate impulses for execution of a program.

Yoga as an Operating system of Life has all the capacity to regulate life force and thus the life, similar to computers. Solar Prān and Lunar Prān within the body are same as '0' and '1' in a computer system. Different permutations and combinations of Prān (Impulses) through Nadis (Circuits) and Chakras (Logical Gates) function similarly as in a computer system to execute a particular program or function.

We shall learn the wisdom of Yoga as our operating system of life to live a Healthy, Happy and Graceful life. It promises the highest technological advancement of mankind that can lead to betterment of the society and the whole Universe.

Today, when human has reached Moon and Mars; life has become fast, furious, effortless and sophisticated; no one will walk a mile if a car is available to one. Human mind has evolved and cultured in this manner. Same is happening with everyone when it comes to Yogic Wisdom for life. They want to learn yoga to help themselves overcome diseases or disorders that hurdles their actions and ambitions without investing much time and efforts. All they need is a quick pill for every problem in their life. If a Yoga guru asks them to perform 'Shavasan' (A Progressive Deep Relaxation Technique of Yoga) or any similar practice that does not fit in their logical mind, they will dissect the essence of the practice rather practicing and experiencing it; as it consumes time and patience of the practitioner. If you dissect a thing, it will not be the same then after nor will it serve your need! So, after my experience for thirty years of Yoga Teaching and Therapy, I have arrived to the conclusion that Yoga shall not only be understood only as a lifelong process or 'Sadhana' as a tool promoting evolution to perfection but an easy, approachable, smart and applicable way to attain sound Physical, Mental, Social and Spiritual health and completeness for today's generation. This quality of modern medicine being an easy, approachable, smart and applicable way to ease (relief) from the sufferings (symptoms) caused by disease without even doing much to cure, has proved the epitome and thus fallaciously has great influence on today's generation. Now a day, time is a constraint. Increased population has created havoc throughout the globe. Everyone is running. Running endlessly, fighting with the constraints of time, fighting with others and the self at the same time. Yoga can serve as a quick pill for aspirants of sound health and also for those who quickly wants to overcome illnesses that are hurdles to their fast and highly ambitious life.

There are so many theories, explanations and understandings about Yoga. Some present it as the Art of Living, some as Indian philosophy, some as Tantra, Some as religion and so on. All may be correct to a certain extent as it is always easy to analyze a given thing through dissecting it or segregating it through similar processes. Structure and composition of the water molecule can easily be known by dissecting it into oxygen and hydrogen, but most difficult to create one. If someone wants to create water, one has to develop a system that works in the same manner and that is developed by Nature as Yoga within an individual for intrinsic cure and balance of life.

Human being is an advanced and highly developed form of Nature's manifestation as life. Human being evolved as an emotional animal that can express feelings and emotions and can laugh, cry, love, care etc. slightly above others that falls in lower categories in animal kingdom. Humans throughout the constant process of evolution have acquired the most from this Yogic wisdom of Nature and started enjoying Nature's bliss.

Wisdom of a race will be lost if not passed on to the descendants as practical knowledge. Something similar happened with the Indian wisdom about inherent wisdom of Yoga and thus elapsed. I am presenting this literature as a part of my endeavor to enlighten everyone on the globe with this inherent wisdom of Yoga as a wisdom of Nature for complete health and intrinsic cure.

I define Yoga thus; "Yoga is the inherent wisdom of a creature to acquire higher levels of evolution to perfection, to live an anticipated life for enjoyment of all the creature comfort offered by Nature and liberate from all bondages (limitations, Diseases, Disorders…) of life".

I have deep faith in this inherent Natural wisdom of

Yoga that has all the capability to prevent and cure almost all the Diseases and Disorders hurdling process of life and evolutionary progress of mankind, if properly understood and explored in a life. May my Gurudev's Blessings bring Health, Joy and utmost Happiness in your Life.

Jay Gurudev.
- Acharya Birju Maharaj

ACHARYA BIRJU MAHARAJ

Yogic Wisdom
YOGNOSIS
Acharya Birju Maharaj

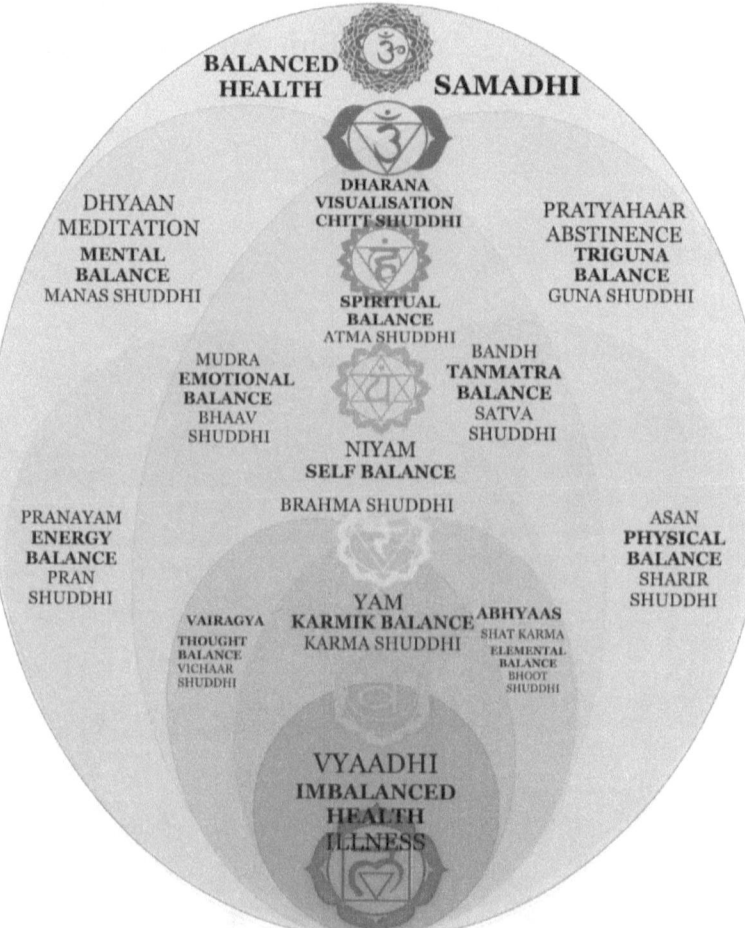

Life is 'Yoga of Nature'

When we draw attention to any system of Prevention and Cure including Yoga, we must first understand Life with all its aspects completely, as any system of cure is pertaining and applied to Life only. Any system that fails to understand life and its aspects cannot correct or cure a Life obviously!

• Nature gives birth to Life with Yoga and maintains it through Yoga. Thus, an individual Life is Yoga of Nature and one needs to understand Nature and Yoga thoroughly to understand Life.

• A Life originates from the union (Yoga) of dual forces within the Nature, Raj (Ovam) (*Prakriti*) and Shukra (Sperm) (*Purush*).

• Main characteristic of Nature is Balance (Samadhi), and so of Yoga and a Life.

• Anything including Life in imbalance cannot survive in Nature. A Life bears all characteristics and follows all the rules and regulations of Nature as an imprint within Genes (Chitt) of an existence.

• Nature has a unique operating system that also work as buffer that helps maintain and bring back the balance. This buffer action within the operating system of Life system is named Yoga. Yoga thus is the common platform for Nature and Life. And can be understood as the Operating system of a computer that is the intermediary between Hardware and Software.

• A Life is an automated system within Nature requires nothing but Natural resources for its creation, existence, reproduction, maintenance, degeneration, evolution and termination.

• A Life is provided all creature comforts by Nature and capable of enjoying the same by the process of evolution through favourably utilizing and updating the operating system of Life (Yoga).

• A human Life bears the most advanced and latest operating system enabling one to enjoy most of Nature's offerings..

• The operating system of Life (Yoga) has all the capabilities to facilitate execution of almost all the programs that governs Life and also protects a Life from imbalances (malware) or Diseases (viruses) those come in the way of its evolution to perfection.

• A Life is the Yoga of Nature, Nature is the Life of Yoga and Yoga is the Nature of Life.

Yoga - The Operating System of Life

It is not difficult to understand the life in its structural (Anatomical) and functional (Physiological) aspects today. One who understands wisdom of Nature (that is based on Binary System) can easily understand the wisdom of Life (Yoga). Nature is Binary in nature. Human Anatomy and Physiology also exist in binary form with different permutations and combinations as of Nature, and also is the same for the entirety of living organisms. One can understand every aspect of life in two opposite vibrating forces that complement each other. 'Yes' or 'No'. 'Functional' or 'non-functional'. 'Living' or 'Dead'. Energy also exists in dual aspect. 'Degenerative' (Catabolic) and 'Regenerative' (Anabolic). That is very similar to the structural composition and functions of computers as seen today. Solar Prān and Lunar Prān within the body are same as '0' and '1' in a computer system. Different permutations and combinations of Prān (Energy) act in response with five basic elements, regulated through Nadis (Circuits) and Chakras (Logical Gates) manifest in a life similarly as done in a computer system to execute a particular program or function. Energy flow throughout the human body through network called Nadis and being regulated through Chakras in the body in a binary flow manner (as done in computers by circuits and logical gates {'AND' and 'NAND' Gate, 'OR' and 'NOR' Gate, 'XOR' and 'XNOR' Gate} which regulate impulses that executes a program).

Thus, Yoga that exists in Nature as the Operating System of Life has all the capacity to regulate life force (energy) that is dual in nature and thus all the aspects of life (similar to a computer program). It is the energy (Impulse) that executes and regulates a life.

There exists third force as the result of play between two opposing complimentary forces manifesting as Sushumnā, Triguṇā, Trivasanā and Incarnation of new life etc.

Sushumnā is the playful manifestation of Idā and Pinglā in equilibrium, Rajas is the meeting point of Satvā and Tamas in Triguṇā s, desire within Trivasanā is the meeting point of need and greed, Incarnation of new life is the assembly of Ojas and Tejas of male and female and so on...

Structure of a Human Body

1. PRAMAN (All those are Verifiable)

Gross Physical/ Structural Body – Panchā Mahabhoot and their various combinations as cell, tissues, organs those build all systems.

Hardware (Mother Board and other physical parts)

2. VIPARYAY (All those are Variable)

Central processing unit: Subtle/Physiological/Functional Body

1. Brain - The seventh top chakra (Sahastrar) with thousand petals.
2. Central Nervous System – Spinal cord – six major Chakras.
3. Autonomic Nervous system – Interplay of Prān with and within Chakras.
4. Circuits: Nerves – Nadis.

3. VIKALP (All those are Discretionary)

Input Devices: (AND–OR, NAND–NOR, XOR–NXOR Gates) Five special senses – Eyes, Ears, Nose, Tongue and Skin.

Output Devices: (AND–OR, NAND–NOR, XOR–NXOR Gates) Five Organs of Function or Action – Arms, Legs, Anus, Mouth and Genitalia.

4. NIDRA (All those are Dormant)

Hard disk: Stored Memory- Storage part of Brain - petals corresponding to Nidra in the top chakra.

5. SMRITI (All those are Accessible) RAM: Random Access Memory- Actively functional part of Brain - petals corresponding to Smriti (RAM) in the top chakra.

Yogic Concept of Health and Illness

Health is defined as 'Samadhi' in Yoga, that literally means Life in a state of Equilibrium at every aspects of it; May it be Physical, Physiological, Emotional, Mental or Spiritual (Atmic) aspects of Life.

Samadhi is the state of Balanced Health of an individual that can be better understood as 'Life in Balance'. Modern sciences call it *Homeostasis* that generally referred as physical and physiological balance only. Thus the word *'Homeostasis'* is a limited concept in modern systems of medicine. Samadhi word covers each aspects of Life and thus is most appropriate.

"Samadhibhavanarthah-
            kleshātanookaranarthashch"-PYS

An objective pursuit of Samadhi (Balanced Health) causes evaporation of Kleshā (Diseases/Disorders).

"Tasya-hetur-avidyā" – PYS

The root cause of kleshās (Diseases) is lack of insight (Avidya).

Root cause of all the Kleshās is Avidhya (Ignorance or lack of insight) about being a yogi who possesses all the capabilities to restrict and cure any Disease or Disorder from within; leads to Asmita (Self Obsession) which further manifest as Raag (Possessiveness) and Dwesh (Isolation) finally surrounds a Life with Abhinivesh (Fear of Unexpected). Fear destroys Wisdom, leading further to the state of Ignorance about self (Avidhya) and the vicious cycle rolls.

When there is proper knowledge and understanding about the operating system of Life (Yoga), that has all the capabilities to confine and cure any diseases or Disorders; one stays in the state of Samadhi (Balanced Health) as Self Obsession, Possessiveness, Segregation and Fear of Unexpected are completely absent.

"Bhava-pratyayo-videha-prakriti-layanam"- P.Y.S.

"Some people are born with true insight (of Nature's wisdom, named Yoga) whereas others attain via a divine body (Guru, who is one with this insight) or oneness with Nature."

None of the creature in Nature needs any medical assistance or external help except human in the world. Amazing! Isn't it? Or is like an antivirus software seller infects the operating systems of others with a self-created virus to satisfy his greed!? May I have hurt many by saying this but is the ultimate truth and all can understand this, obviously!

All system of cure started providing assistance with

processes of Natural Healing and we all know where they are heading today!? I do not point any particular system of cure but all. When Vidhya (Knowledge) about the Nature and the self (Being Yogi) can confine and cure any Diseases or Disorders, what are we doing towards this Gnosis or Salvation?

'Bhavtapen-taptanam, Yogohi paramaushadhah' - Upanishad.

Meaning: Yoga is the only cure for those who suffer from (Trividh Tāp) all worldly grievances (Adhi, Vyadhi and Upadhi). Explanation of that is- "Yoga is the only cure for all worldly sufferings and distresses."

Yogic Lore in Health and Illness (Yognosis)

Yogic Lore had been identified by yognostics of Hind (India) and cultured in the roots of all Indians as lifestyle to empower them with Vim, Vigour and Vitality that can offer a great sense of health, bliss and also the ability to prevent and also to cure if there manifests any imbalances, diseases or disorders. No wonder, people in India enjoyed great health and self-confidence till systems of medicine were introduced! When a pill can cure symptoms or when a fractured bone can be set right without pain, who cares for the cause or Natural remedy? This mind set of people has caused irreparable damage to the society at large. People forgot about their own responsibility to keep healthy and cure themselves naturally and eventually became totally dependent on such systems of medicines even for cough and cold!? Ayurveda, a rich system of longevity and cure was immerged when man-made diseases started prevailing and those preceded with permanence; and helped people stay healthy and illness-free when people forgot to live Natural Yogic Lifestyle. Ayurveda is an extention of Yogic Wisdom and shares a single platform with Yoga in almost all the aspects of life, knowledge and wisdom; eventually got identified as a separate system of medicine as it used some herbs and their concoctions with or without some alloys and improvised material methods of Panchkarmas over Yogic Shatkarmas and surgeries to cure diseases which falls under limitations of Yogic Lore. Ayurveda also offers a great remedy for God-made diseases like Natural calamities, accidents, trauma, surgery and genetically inherited diseases and thus plays an important role as an adjuvant system of cure with Yoga if one fails to observe healthy Yogic Lifestyle or a complete cure from a Yognostic (A Yoga Therapist of Yogic Lore) and surrounds oneself with diseases, mostly for those preceded with permanence as Kleshāyukt Chitt Samskar (Genetic manifestation in the progeny as a disease). Modern medicine is a further extension of Ayurveda as panacea and started using synthetic drugs over Natural ones, chemicals over herbal concoctions and synthetic bio-chemicals. Stem-cell and gene therapies with a great idea to overcome limitations of Ayurveda but seems to have completely lost the basic idea and is now headed towards highly hazardous, costly, life threatening counterfeit practice by some greedy people running healthcare industries.

None of the Gnostic or physician intend to expertise in their respective practices to rob or mislead the patient but industry! All of them start their learning and practice in the field of health care with a great intention to help and cure the diseased. It is the people in the industry with greed forcefully mould them in their malefic frame.

To enroot this inherent wisdom of Nature called Yoga in a Life, wise selected a subconscious route as found it difficult to make common people understand and accept the same and cultured Yogic Lifestyle wrapped in a spiritual enigma of temple and the deities. They were so wise that this way they made all understand and follow the wisdom of Yoga and its significance in life without being questioned or obstructed by logical and rational minds who always ask for evidences!

Some of the awesome presentations of Yogic wisdom

in Indian Mythological Scriptures for practical applications to healthy, joyous and blissful life are explained in this section below.

It is really surprising to know that the precise facts about Life are seeded in the scriptures. And the fact is even more surprising then that is to a common man. In my constant Endeavour to unravel the acumen behind these presentations of Indian wisdom of Yoga with the blessings and directions of my Guru, I have tried to simplify the wisdom of Yoga to people for better understanding.

It is well established fact that the life is directed and determined by sub-conscious, super conscious and cosmic mind many a fold more than the conscious mind. The knowledge to the sub-conscious, super conscious and cosmic mind is only the key to lead its practical manifestation for better life.

Realizing the need to develop these occult wisdom as deeper sub-conscious and super conscious wisdom and to avoid impractical logical conflicts, Gnostics (Seers and Rishis) of India have presented same in the form of spiritual mythological stories to the world. The story of Lord Śiva and Goddess Śakti.

Lord Śiva the AdiYogi (a realised individual), as described by the scriptures, was staying at 'Kailās' – the mount in Himalayās, and Goddess Śakti (Pārvati-Kundalini) in the valley of Himalayās. This is the presentation of the Agya Chakra sitting on the peak ('Kailās') of pyramidal body of Śiva (Resembling a Mountain) sitting on the 'Kailās' (Agya Chakra) controlling the life and Kundalini Śakti (Pārvati) at the base (valley) constantly empowering herself to reach the Agya chakra through regulation of Prānic flow. They meet each other by tireless efforts of Pārvati (Kundalini Śakti) known as 'Tapascharya' (KriyaYoga- Tap, Swadhyay and IshwarPrānidhan). The meeting of the two deities is thrilling and full of romance that is same as practiced and experienced by Yogis at union of Kundalini Śakti with Agya Chakra. The result is the reincarnation through transformation of these energies (Tejas and Ojas) into Mooladhara (Lord Ganesha) and Anahata (Lord Kartikeya) controlling Apāna and Prān- The basic vayus responsible to regulate and maintain life. Lord Ganesha is sitting at Mooladhara Chakra as the protector of Kundalini Śakti (Mother Pārvati) preventing aliens including Lord Śiva to enter the place when she is bathing or say having showers of vigour from Swadhishthana Chakra to empower herself to reach to Agya Chakra (Lord Śiva). Okha being the Sushumnā Nadi gets dissolved in the BrahmNadi when Lord Śiva (Agya Chakra) is excited to facilitate his meeting with Pārvati (Kundalini Śakti). Lord Kartikeya revolves around in the whole body as Prān Vayu but limited to create any impact on Śiva and Pārvati as Ganesha does by facilitating the meeting through energizing the Kundalini Śakti (Mother Pārvati) to enter the 'BrahmNadi' through the desired route. It is thus described that, Lord Ganesha will stay on the entrance of the Temple of Lord Śiva and Pārvati and will be prayed first before entering to the temple similarly as described in Yogic Anatomy and Physiology.

Having described the qualities, place, roles and powers of deities, 'Rishis' have invoked the power of sub-conscious mind to grasp and practically execute the knowledge of qualities, place, roles and powers of organs and systems (Kundalini, Chakras and Nadis) of Human body and it's Anatomy and Physiology at deeper levels for its sub-conscious practical implementation in day to day life for health, happiness and harmony without exercising the compulsion for conscious efforts.

Many a times a person experiences the divine help at many situations. This divine help is nothing but the help of the sixth sense developed in an individual through sub-conscious and super conscious mind. Our seers and 'rishis' having the utmost knowledge and wisdom of life, have presented Yogic wisdom of life wrapped in mystic mythological stories with a view to equip one with this ultimate wisdom at the deeper levels of sub-conscious and super conscious mind.

Applied Yoga – Yoga Therapy (Core)

It is really insane to find remedy after destructions being done! All the systems of medicine are limited to their application after onset of symptoms and diagnosis of a disease. These limitations of systems of medicine other than Yoga thus fail to prevent any disease effectively. The only system of medicine on this Planet offers prevention of diseases or disorders and that is Yoga. The simplest, affordable for all, non-hazardous, intrinsic and non-invasive system of medicine namely Yoga, is still struggling to hold the position of primary system of medicine!? Yoga must be freed from prejudices and doubts.

Aim of any therapy or system of cure should be,

1. To help sustain sound health of the healthy and Prevent Disease and Disorders.

2. To take away fear of the diseased to facilitate inherent cure.

3. To eradicate root cause of illness completely and not keeping patient in disease by merely suppressing symptoms.

4. Healing is within. To allow natural and inherent healing to cure one before starting any other remedies unless the condition is a life threatening trauma. Any path of treatment is 'faith healing' as healing is within and a patient's own will and systems are responsible for healing and not merely the supportive medicines and a practitioner of any therapy should not lose faith of the patient on him.

Though regular practice of Yoga assures complete health and cure for almost all the chronic diseases, majority of people still are resistant to adopt this supreme inherent natural divine practice!?

Let me give some of the reasons why Yoga is bound with unnecessary doubts and prejudices.

1. People over the period of time have been forced and mislead with so called research work and documentation of the same. No doubt about research work done in the field of Yoga as Therapy till date, but the question is that, are researchers on a right tract? Does research methods applied satisfies all the principles of the system being researched? Not yet. There are no analytical systems developed till date those can measure emotions, individual perceptions, belief system, memories, social status and limitations, spiritual status, racial characteristics,

genetic adaptations, natural resistance etc.

2. The lucid belief system of modern medicine that is widespread today fails to understand the basic healing principles of Yoga, keeps it on the opposite pole; While Yoga should be their primary preference.

3. People refuse to believe that which is not observable. For example, people never believed and misunderstood the word 'bhoot' (a name given to microorganisms in India at a time when those were not visible) causing disease but started believing the same as micro-organisms or pathogens after seeing it under microscope, even knowing the fact that microscopes does not show pathogenesity of such organisms!? According to people, Prān (Life Force), Chakras, Nadis, Kundalini etc. does not exist, as is not observable or varifiable.

4. A huge gap between Yoga and modern system of medicine is not natural but induced by some materialistic people. Despite the fact that Yoga is primary system that fundamentally helps all other systems of cure.

5. Today, human has reached Moon and Mars; life has become fast, furious, effortless and sophisticated; no one will walk a mile if a car is available to one. Human mind has evolved and cultured in this manner. Same is happening with everyone when it comes to Yogic Wisdom for life.

Cycles of Prānic energy (Life force) in a Life

Daily cycle of Prān in Chakras

- Day time from Sun rise to Sun set Prānic energy pervades and dominates as Tejas, flowing downwards from Sahastrar to Mooladhar.

- Night time from Sun set to Sun Rise Prānic energy pervades and dominates as Ojas, flowing upwards from Mooladhar to Sahastrar.

- Energy is utilized as Tejas in the day time while gets accumulated as Ojas in the Night.

- There are two times when energy is Stable. Not flowing upwards or downwards. Those are Brahmamuhurta (Morning 4 to 6 am) and Sandhya (Evening 4 to 6 pm). In Brahmamuhurta, there is abundant amount of Ojas as acquired and stored during night at rest and at Sandhya there is diminished amount of Ojas as spent by activities that utilizes Tejas. The less Ojas is spent as Tejas during the day in activities or the more Ojas acquired during night, the more is energy, longevity and health of the being. Human breathes approximately 21600 breathes in 24 hours.

Time and Energy cycle	Chakra	Number of Breathes
4 to 6 am – Brahmamuhurta - Neutral	Sahastrar	1000 breathes
6 to 8 am Tejas and 2 to 4 am Ojas	Agya	1000 breathes
8 to 10 Tejas am and 12 to 2 am Ojas	Vishuddhi	1000 breathes
10 am to 12 pm Tejas and 10 pm to 12 am Ojas	Anahat	6000 breathes
12 to 2 pm Tejas and 8 to 10 pm Ojas	Manipur	6000 breathes
2 to 4 pm Tejas and 6 to 8 pm Ojas	Swadhishthan	6000 breathes
4 to 6 pm - Sandhya - Neutral	Mooladhar	600 breathes

As described in table above, Prān Travels downward from Sahastrar to Mooladhar in the Day time (Catabolism-degeneration) while upwards from Mooladhar to Sahastrar in Night (Anabolism-regeneration). During its upward movement it fills the chakra with Ojas Prān and during downward movement it uses acquired Ojas Prān to support the activity of the Tejas Prān.

Monthly Cycle of Prān in Chakras

Month wise Prānic dominance	Chakra	Prān Type
16th December to 15th January	Sahastrar	Neutral
16th January to 15th February	Agya	Ojas.
16th February to 15th March	Vishuddhi	Tejas
16th March to 15th April	Anahat	Ojas
16th April to 15th May	Manipur	Tejas
16th May to 15th June	Swadhishthan	Ojas
16th June to 15th July	Mooladhaar	Neutral
16th July to 15 August	Swadhishthan	Ojas
16th August to 15th September	Manipur	Tejas
16th September to 15th October	Anahat	Ojas
16th October to 15th November	Vishuddhi	Tejas
16th November to 15th December	Agya	Ojas

Life cycle of Prān in Chakras

Nature has designed a growth and degenerative cycle of human life in multiples of 7 yrs.

The Śakti cycle of Prān

Age-Years	Dominant Chakra	Role of Prānic energy
0 to 7 years	Mooladhaar	Happiness, Stability, Weight Gain, Vim, Fearlessness And Zest for Life.
8 to 14 years	Swadhishthan	Boosting Up Sex Hormones, Lust, Vigour, Beauty, Creativity, Attraction, Inspiration.
15 to 21 years	Manipur	Elevating Higher Ambitions, Aggression, Increased Appetite, Vitality, Self-Confidence, Abilities, Ego, Desire to Conquer World.
22 to 28 years	Lower Anahat	Expansions Of Family, Greed, Care, Togetherness, Creed And Transformation From Individual Being To Universal Being.
29 to 36 years	Anahat	Expansions Of Self, Unconditional Love, Forgiveness, Vitality And Oneness.

37 to 42 years	Vishuddhi	Loud Self-Expression, Accreditation And Acknowledgement Of Work Done, Transparency, Emotional Surge, Seeking Truth, Demonstrations of Acquired Abilities.
43 to 49 years	Agya	Balancing Emotions, Expectations, Limitations, Abilities And Self Realization.
50 to 56 years	Sahastrar	To Realize Act Of God (Nature) That Each One Is Mortal And Degeneration Will Start No Sooner And Aspiration For Doing Something To Leave Great Impression On World About Self, Universal Consciousness And Ecstasy.

From the age 0 to 56 there is regenerative Śakti cycle.

From the age 56 to 112 there will be degenerative Śiva (Roodra) cycle of life.

• First seven years after birth, Prānic energy explores in and energizes Mooladhar chakra ensuring happiness, stability, weight gain, fearlessness and zest for life.

• From 8 to 14 Prānic energy explores in and energizes swadhishthan chakra boosting up sex hormones, lust, vigour, beauty, creativity, attraction and inspiration.

• From 15 to 21 Prānic energy explores in and energises Manipur Chakra elevating higher ambitions, aggression, increased appetite, self-confidence, capability, ego, desire to conquer world.

- From 22 to 28 Prānic energy explores in and energises lower Anahat Chakra promoting expansions of Family, greed, care, togetherness, creed and transformation from individual being to universal being.

- From 29 to 36 Prānic energy explores in and energises Anahat chakra promoting expansions of self, unconditional love, forgiveness, Vitality and oneness.

- From 37 to 42 Prānic energy explores in and energizes Vishuddhi Chakra leading one to loud self-expression, accreditation and acknowledgement of work done, transparency, emotional surge, seeking truth and demonstrations of acquired abilities.

- From 43 to 49 Prānic energy explores in and energizes Agya Chakra balancing emotions, expectations, limitations, abilities and self realization.

- From 49 to 56 in Sahastrar chakra leading one to realize acts of God (Nature) that each one is mortal and degeneration will start no sooner and aspiration for doing something to leave great impression on world about self, universal consciousness and ecstasy.

Then starts degenerative Śiva cycle of Prān in life...

Planets, Chakras and Effect.

Graha (Planet)	Chakra	Effect
Universal Surya (SUN) as Hiranya Garbh	Sahastrar	Chetna (Chitt/Genes) (Source of Creation)
Chandra (MOON)	Agya	Manas (Mind)
Guru (JUPITER)	Vishuddhi	Gyanendriyas (Special Senses)
Shani (SATURN)	Anahat	Karmendriyas (Senses of Action)
Budh (MERCURY)	Lower Anahat	Buddhi (Intellect)
Inner Surya (SUN)	Manipur	Ahamkar (Ego) (Basic Instincts)
Shukra (VENUS)	Swadhishthan	Trivaasana (Need, Desire and Greed)
Mangal (MARS)	Mooladhaar	Triguna (Satva, Rajas and Tamas)

YOGIC VIEW OF BODY

- **COSMIC BODY** — BRAHMAND SHARIR
- **GROSS BODY** — STHOOL SHARIR / ANNAMAYA KOSH
- **SUBTLE BODY** — SUKSHMA SHARIR
  - **ENERGY BODY** — PRANMAYA KOSH
  - **BIOCHEMICAL BODY** — VIGYANMAYA KOSH
  - **PSYCHIC BODY** — MANOMAYA KOSH
- **CAUSAL BODY** — CHITT / ANANDMAYA KOSH

AVIDHYA
LACK OF KNOWLEDGE
IGNORANCE ABOUT TRUE SELF

ASMITA
EGO CENTRICITY

RAAG
ATTACHMENT

ABHINIVESH
FEAR OF UNCERTAINITY

DWESH
HATRED

VYADHI
DISEASE/DISORDER

YOGIC VIEW OF ILLNESS

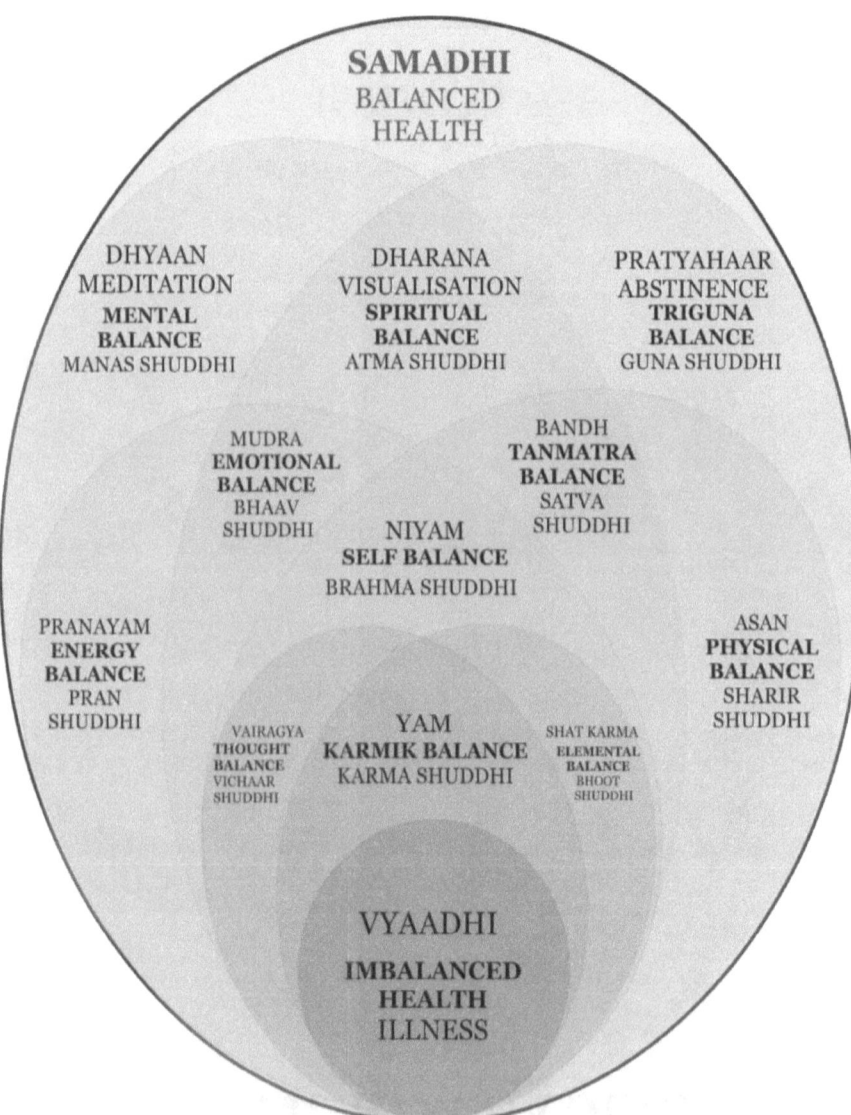

YOGIC PATHWAY - FROM ILLNESS TO HEALTH

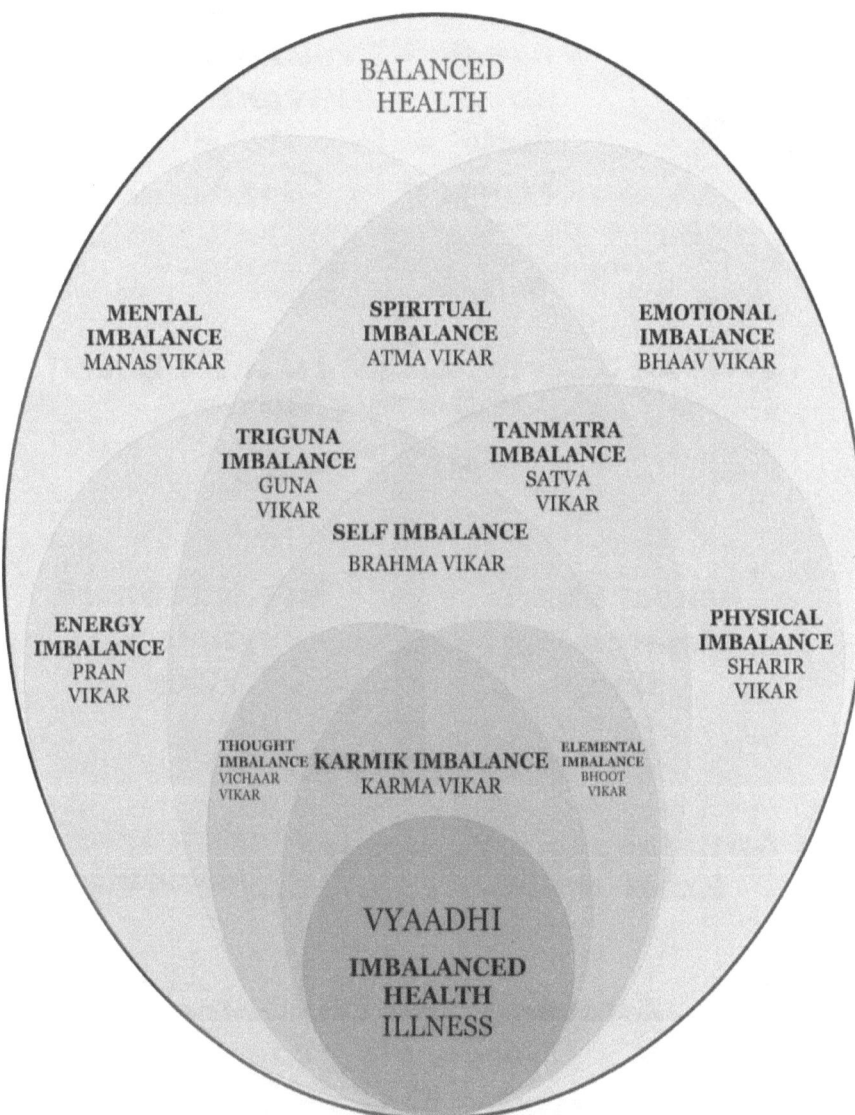

YOGIC PATHWAY - FROM HEALTH TO ILLNESS

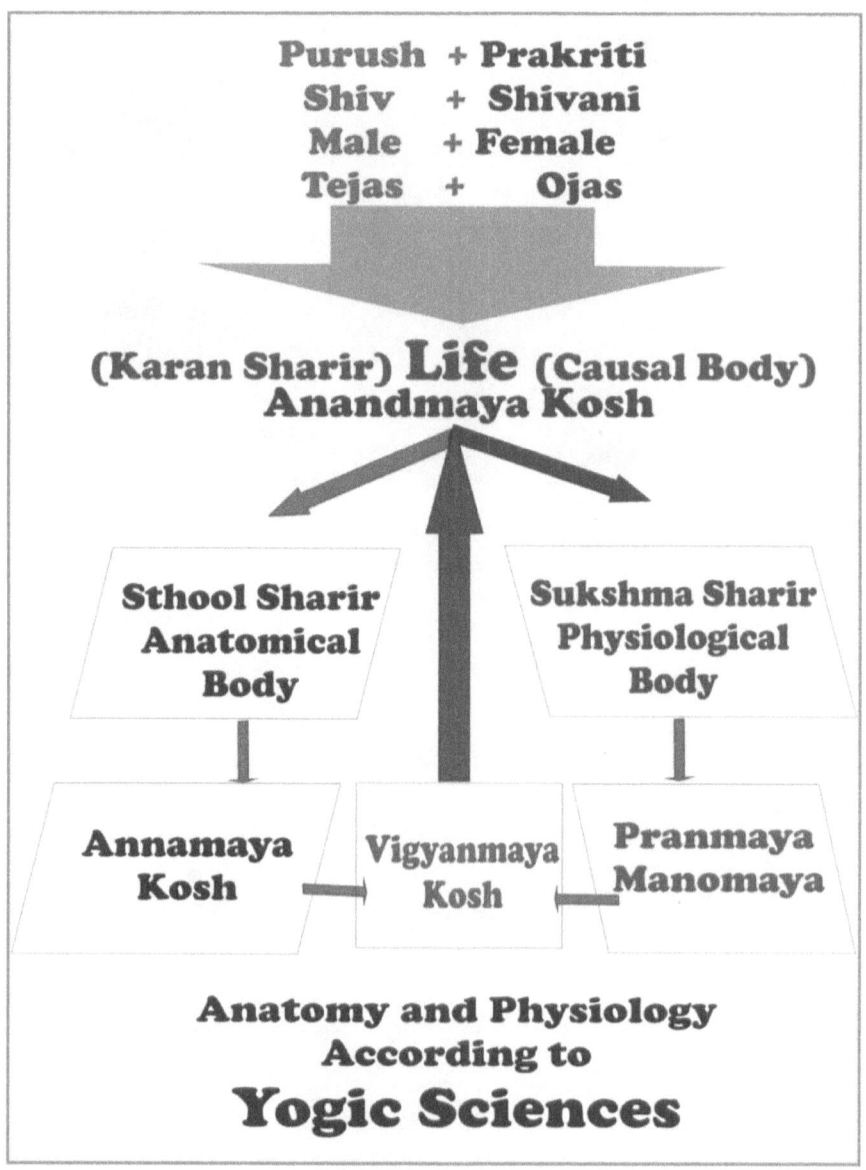

Disease according to Yoga

Any imbalance in Samadhi state of body, mind, intellect and spirit leading to physical, mental, emotional or spiritual imbalances is termed as Vyadhi or Kleshā (Disease) according to Yoga.

There are only two types of Kleshās (Diseases) and that are

1) Man-made (Caused due to Avidhya) and

2) God-made (Nature's exasperation)

And each of which have two aspects:
1. **Somatic and 2. Psychosomatic**
   Further can be divided into 4 stages and those are
   1. **Dormant (Prasupt)**
   2. **Developing (Tanu)**
   3. **Developed (Vichchhina)**
   4. **Devastating (Udaar).**

1) Man-made Vyadhis (Diseases) are the imbalances caused by human beings, may it be somatic or psychosomatic. Man-made diseases are caused by Avidhya causing improper postures, breathing, Sleep, dietary and other living habits, unnatural individual perceptions and emotional imbalances, wrongful imposition of a disease by self or physicians, wrong influences and predominant ignorance about the inherent wisdom of healing process initiated and completed by Nature through Yoga.

2) God (Nature)-made Vyadhis (Diseases) are the disharmony caused due to imbalances in Nature. Most of the times induced by Natural calamities, Epidemics, Irregularities, Seasons and sometimes of inheritance (Genetic origin).

To be Continued in part – 2………

Narayan….Narayan…. Narayan…..Narayan…..

ABOUT THE AUTHOR

Acharya Birju Maharaj is a traditional Yognostic from a affluent Yoga Tradition and direct disciple of Sami Manuvaryaji Maharaj. His life is dedicated to extend the Indian ancestral wisdom of Yoga to the world, as of his Guruji. He is practicing as Yoga Mentor and Therapist from 1988 and is devoted to see that Wisdom of Yoga benefit all in the world.

www.ingramcontent.com/pod-product-compliance
Lightning Source LLC
Chambersburg PA
CBHW030513220526
45464CB00006B/2779